HEADLINE ISSUES

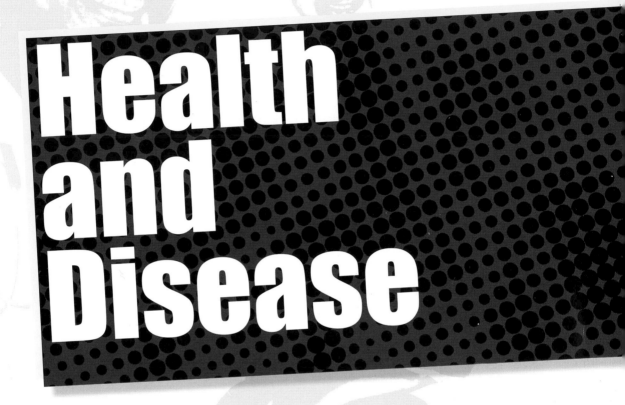

Health and Disease

Sarah Levete

Raintree is an imprint of Capstone Global Library
Limited, a company incorporated in England and Wales
having its registered office at 7 Pilgrim Street, London,
EC4V 6LB - Registered company number: 6695582

Raintree is a registered trademark of Pearson Education
Limited, under licence to Capstone Global Library
Limited

Text © Capstone Global Library Limited 2009
First published in hardback in 2009
Paperback edition first published in 2010
The moral rights of the proprietor have been asserted.

Edited by Sarah Eason and Leon Gray
Designed by Calcium and Geoff Ward
Original illustrations © Capstone Global Library
Limited 2009
Illustrated by Geoff Ward
Picture research by Maria Joannou
Originated by Heinemann Library
Printed and bound in China by CTPS

ISBN 978 0 431162 77 5 (hardback)
13 12 11 10 09
10 9 8 7 6 5 4 3 2 1

ISBN 978 0 431162 89 8 (paperback)
14 13 12 11 10
10 9 8 7 6 5 4 3 2 1

British Library Cataloguing in Publication Data
Levete, Sarah
Health and disease. - (Headline issues)
362.1
A full catalogue record for this book is available from the
British Library.

Acknowledgements
We would like to thank the following for permission to
reproduce photographs:
Alamy Images: Eye Ubiquitous 28t, Imagebroker 7,
Images of Africa Photobank 13; Corbis: Howard Davies
27, Wang Haiyan/China Features 25, Ahmed Jallanzo/
EPA 9t; Fotolia: Cynthia Chung 18–19; Getty Images:
Peter Essick 9b, Jean-Marc Giboux 22, Andrew Wong
20; Istockphoto: Carmen Martínez Banús 14, Pathathai
Chungyam 4, 5, Ralph125 19, Patrick Roherty 16–17, 16,
Catherine Yeulet 28b; Public Health Image Library:
James Gathany 10; Rex Features: Burger/Phanie 24, Peter
Oxford/Nature Picture Library 11, F Sierakowski 18,
Sipa Press 21; Science Photo Library: James Cavallini 5,
Andy Crump/TDR/WHO 12; Shutterstock: 3777190317
20–21, AJT 22–23, Keith Brook 25, Jacek Chabraszewski
30–31, Ivan Cholakov 10–11, Stephen Coburn 4, Matthew
Collingwood 14, Lucian Coman 20, Jaimie Duplass 23,
Peter Elvidge 26, ENE 15, Gelpi 1, 23, Eric Isselée 12,
Sebastian Kaulitzki 24–25, Muriel Lasure 17, Jon Le-
Bon 6, MaszaS 28–29, Dmitry Matrosov 17, MaxPhoto
6, Laurin Rinder 26–27, Salamanderman 8, Maksim
Shmeljov 26, Liudmila P. Sundikova 18, Tkachuk 12–13,
Kheng Guan Toh 32, Miroslav Tolimir 4, Valentyn Volkov
3, Mark Winfrey 8–9, Wojciech Wojcik 10; Still Pictures:
Adrian Arbib 7.

Cover photograph reproduced with permission of Getty
Images/Jean-Marc Giboux.

Every effort has been made to contact copyright holders
of material reproduced in this book. Any omissions will
be rectified in subsequent printings if notice is given to
the publishers.

Disclaimer
All the Internet addresses (URLs) given in this book
were valid at the time of going to press. However, due to
the dynamic nature of the Internet, some addresses may
have changed, or sites may have changed or ceased to
exist since publication. While the author and Publishers
regret any inconvenience this may cause readers, no
responsibility for any such changes can be accepted by
either the author or the Publishers.

Contents

Some words are printed in bold, **like this**. You can find out what they mean by looking in the glossary on page 30.

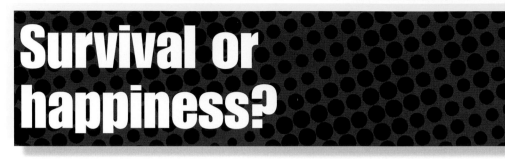

Survival or happiness?

WHAT DOES HEALTH mean to you? It may mean feeling fit and well, or it may mean feeling happy. For others, health means being able to enjoy a full and rewarding life. For many of the world's poorest people, health means simply survival.

Today, doctors have a detailed understanding of how to treat illness. They can **prescribe** people medicines to make them better. However, in some parts of the world people cannot afford to see a doctor. A child in a rich, **developed country** can have an operation to cure an eye problem. In a poor, **developing country**, the same child would go blind. Many people in the developing world cannot even afford to see a doctor.

All in the mind

Health is not just to do with physical wellbeing. Mental health is the way people feel about themselves.

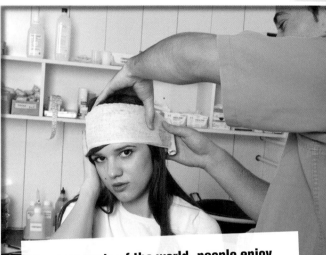

In some parts of the world, people enjoy healthy lives. They can see doctors when they need to and do not have to worry about finding enough food to eat.

Many people suffer from mental health problems. These affect how people behave and their moods. Most of these problems can be treated with support from doctors and counsellors and sometimes with drugs. Many people with mental health problems continue living and working as usual.

FACT!

◆ In Japan, a person can on average expect to live to about 82 years of age.
◆ In Mozambique, a person can on average expect to live to about 41 years of age.

BEHIND THE HEADLINES
Getting to grip with germs

Germs are everywhere. These tiny living things are on your hands, on tables, on food, and in the air. There are many different types of germs. They include **bacteria** and **viruses**. Some germs are friendly but others cause deadly diseases. You can only see germs by looking at them through a machine called a **microscope**.

This is a close-up of the virus that causes a disease called influenza (or flu).

Dying of poverty

POVERTY MEANS NOT having enough money for basic items such as shelter, food, and clean water. Millions of people around the world are dying because they don't have enough money for these essential things. These people are more likely to catch diseases, because they live in poor conditions and drink dirty water.

Failing crops

In the developing world, people often grow their own food to feed their families and sell some of it to earn money. When **crops** fail, perhaps because of a severe drought or flood, the family goes without food. There is also no money to buy medicine.

Poverty in rich countries

People are suffering in many parts of the developed world, too. Many people do not have enough money. Some have nowhere to live. Without a home, they cannot find work to earn money. People get trapped in a cycle of poverty. Homeless people sleep on the streets without any shelter from bad weather. They also find it difficult to find food. Many homeless people become sick without these essential items.

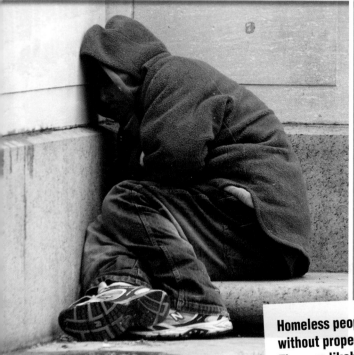

Homeless people sleep on the streets without proper shelter and enough food. They are likely to become very ill.

FACT!
- ✦ Half the world – more than three billion people – live in poverty.
- ✦ More than 26,000 children die every day due to the effects of poverty.

ON THE SPOT

Vietnam

A family gathers to eat at their home in a mountain village in Vietnam. Wood burns on a small fire. Like many others, this family can only afford to burn wood or coal. There is no chimney, so the smoke clogs up the small house. The family uses the fire to cook and to heat the home in the chilly evenings.

The children have breathing difficulties. Their mother, who does most of the cooking in the kitchen, keeps coughing. The fumes from the smoke are harmful and **pollute** the air. Other fuels are less polluting but more expensive. The family cannot afford a stove with a chimney to get rid of the smoke.

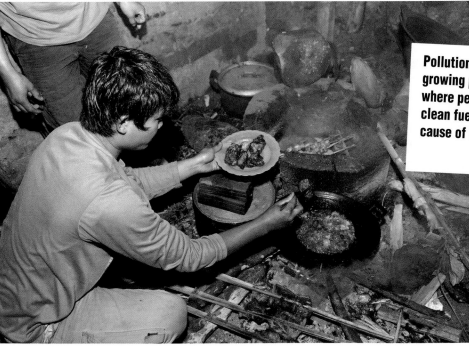

Pollution in the home is a growing problem in countries where people cannot afford clean fuels. It is a major cause of ill health.

No food and dirty water

PEOPLE CANNOT LIVE without water and food. However, dirty water and **malnutrition** (caused by a lack of food) can also kill. People become very weak when they do not have enough to eat. This can affect growth and development and makes it hard to fight off disease. Drawing fresh, clean water from wells and having simple, clean toilets can mean the difference between life and death.

Dirty water

People from some **developing countries** do not have freshwater. They often walk miles to fill up buckets with water from a river or lake. Often animals drink from these rivers and lakes. Raw **sewage** may also be in the water. The water is often infected with **germs** that cause serious diseases such as **cholera** and dysentry, a severe infection of the digestive system.

Cholera

Cholera strikes where there is no clean drinking water. The disease causes severe vomiting and diarrhoea. People lose a lot of fluid and become **dehydrated**. They need special drugs to replace the lost fluids and treat the cholera. Drinking clean water can also help. In the developing world, there is usually no clean water to drink and no drugs available.

Dirty food

A **bacterium** called *Escherichia coli* lives in the body and keeps us healthy. However, some types of *E. coli* cause disease. They are found in meat that is not cooked properly or vegetables that have been grown with manure. Washing hands after using the toilet and before preparing food can help stop the spread of *E. coli*.

✦ Around 1.2 billion people in developing countries do not have access to clean water.

✦ Every day, 4,000 children die from a water-related disease.

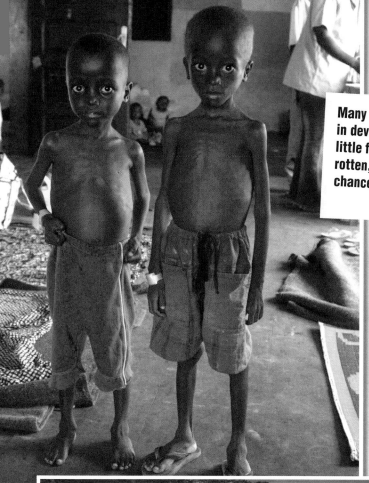

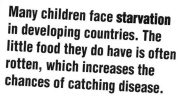

Many children face **starvation** in developing countries. The little food they do have is often rotten, which increases the chances of catching disease.

Animal droppings in the water may contain germs. Sharing the same water that animals use can easily spread disease.

Spreading disease

WHY DO PEOPLE cover their mouths when they cough or sneeze? The simple answer is to stop **germs** from spreading. For the same reason, you wash your hands after using the toilet. Illnesses that spread from person to person are called **communicable diseases**.

Some illnesses spread in the air, and others in water and food. Some animals can spread disease. Insects often pick up germs from waste such as poo. The insects then land on food, leaving the germs behind. A person can then become ill if they eat the infected food.

Travel brings disease

More people are visiting foreign countries. People take their germs with them when they travel. **Infectious** diseases that once remained in one country are now appearing in different parts of the world. A person carrying a disease may have a natural protection against the germ that causes it. Others may not be so lucky.

Killer insects

In many African countries, mosquitoes carry the germs that cause a disease called **malaria**. Only the female mosquitoes can pass on the disease. They usually bite people between sunset and sunrise.

Malaria is one of the world's biggest killers. Many people suffer from this disease. One thing everyone can do to stop getting bitten is to use a mosquito net sprayed with **insecticide**. This is a chemical that keeps the mosquitoes away.

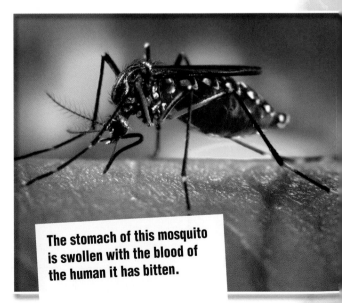

The stomach of this mosquito is swollen with the blood of the human it has bitten.

✦ Each year between 350 and 500 million cases of malaria occur worldwide.
✦ More than 1 million people die from malaria each year. Most of them are children.

ON THE SPOT
Cumerjali, Peru

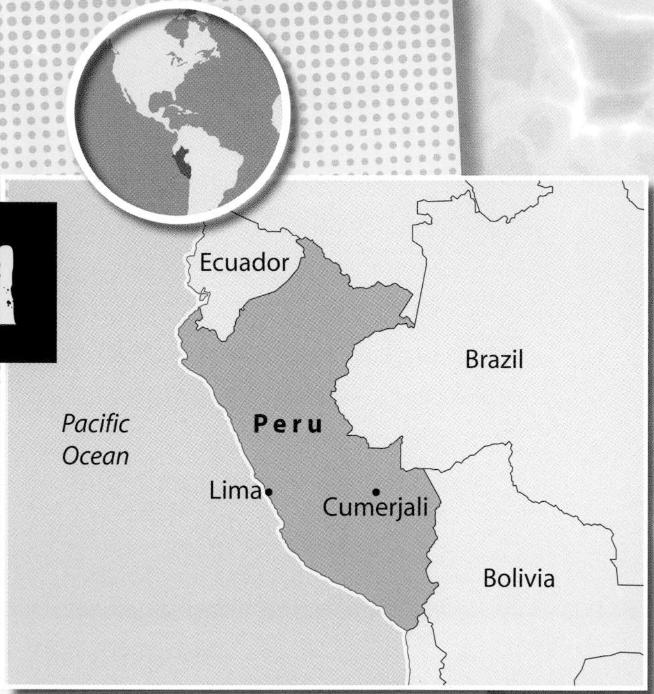

In the remote area of Cumerjali in Peru, several groups of native or indigenous people live traditional lives. They have no contact with the rest of the world. They have never been in contact with the germs that cause colds or the flu. When tourists or other people enter these communities, they bring their germs with them. The native people have no natural protection against these germs. A simple cold may kill and destroy a whole community.

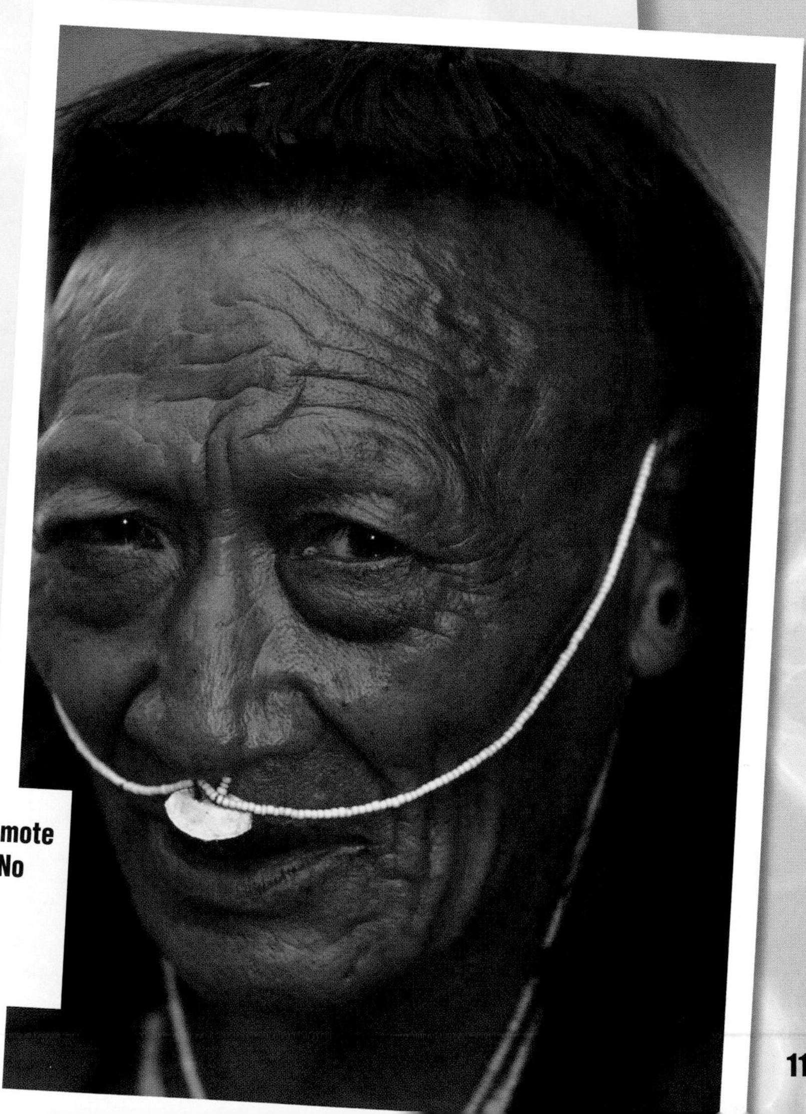

Ecuador

Brazil

Pacific
Ocean

P e r u

Lima•

•Cumerjali

Bolivia

The Yaminahua people live in remote parts of the Amazon rainforest. No one knew about the Yaminahua people until 1988.

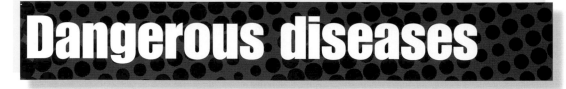

Dangerous diseases

COMMUNICABLE DISEASES ARE more dangerous in **developing countries**, where there are often no toilets and no clean supplies of freshwater. **Germs** can spread quickly in dirty water.

In the **developed world**, people tend to suffer more from diseases such as heart disease and **cancer**.

You cannot catch heart disease. People develop heart disease through poor lifestyle choices. These include being overweight, not taking enough exercise, smoking cigarettes, drinking too much alcohol, and eating unhealthy foods rich in fat and sugar.

An old killer returns

Tuberculosis, or TB for short, is on the rise again. TB is caused by **bacteria** that attack the lungs and other parts of the body. If left untreated, TB can kill. In fact, it has been a killer disease for thousands of years.

TB bacteria have been found in the preserved bodies, or mummies, of the ancient Egyptians who lived thousands of years ago. In the middle of the 20th century, modern medicines helped to get rid of TB. Today, it has made an unwelcome return and is killing millions of people around the world. Some strains or types of TB are becoming very difficult to treat with drugs.

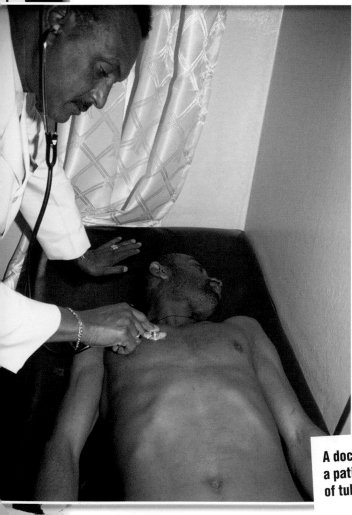

A doctor listens to the lungs of a patient for the telltale signs of tuberculosis infection.

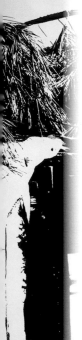

BEHIND THE HEADLINES
The body goes to war

When germs invade the body, the **immune system** fights back. The body is made up of billions of tiny structures called **cells**. When germs enter the body, cells from the immune system start to attack the germs. A person becomes ill if the immune system cannot fight the germs. Children, pregnant women, and the elderly are more at risk from some diseases. Their immune systems are not as strong or fully developed as those of healthy adults.

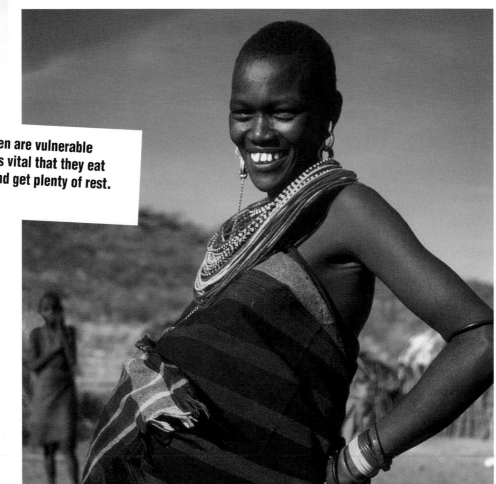

Pregnant women are vulnerable to disease. It is vital that they eat healthy food and get plenty of rest.

Animal killers

Some diseases pass between animals and people. Some of these diseases may be linked to the way we produce food.

Mad cows

During the 1980s, some farmers in Britain noticed that their cattle were behaving strangely. The cows had a brain disease called bovine spongiform encephalopathy (BSE), for which there is no cure. They had been fed with food made from the bones and brains of other animals. BSE is more commonly called "mad cow disease". A rare form of BSE, called Creutzfeldt-Jakob disease (CJD), can be passed on to people.

Today, cattle are not given food made from animal products such as meat or bone. Some countries do not allow meat from British cattle into their countries.

Mad dogs

Bats, cats, dogs, and foxes can carry a dangerous disease called rabies. People can catch rabies if they are bitten by an infected animal. About 30 countries are free from rabies. They operate strict controls to prevent infected animals from entering their country. In other countries, between 30,000 and 50,000 people are killed by rabies each year.

Some scientists think that people can catch CJD by eating beef from BSE-infected cows. Between 1990 and 2008, more than 1,300 people died from the human form of mad cow disease.

BEHIND THE HEADLINES
Bird flu

In 1997, a three-year-old boy was killed by flu. He had caught a particular type of flu from an infected bird. Since then, more than 200 people have died from this "bird flu". Experts think that the disease first spread in parts of Asia. In some countries, chickens and ducks often live in close contact with humans, in basic conditions.

This is how scientists believe the bird flu spread from an animal to a person. There is little evidence to suggest that people can catch the disease from bird meat. However, scientists are worried that bird flu will soon pass from human to human. This may cause a worldwide outbreak, or **epidemic**, of this dangerous disease.

Healthy turkeys are at risk of catching bird flu as the disease becomes more common.

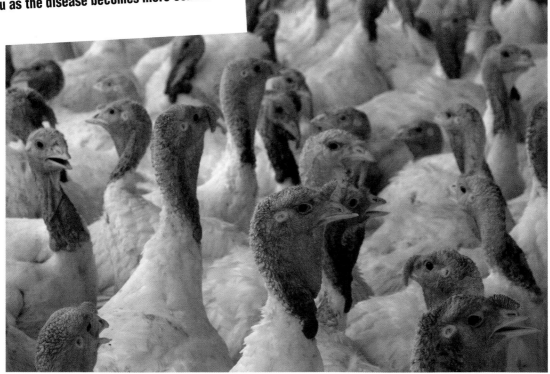

Growing cities spread disease

WHERE YOU LIVE has a great impact on your health. It's not just **poverty** in the countryside that kills people.

Mosquitoes on the move

Every year, huge areas of forest are cut down. Deforestation clears the land for new **crops** and new houses. It also has a big effect on people's health. Insects adapt to different **environments**. Mosquitoes that once thrived in tree hollows adapt to live in **sewage** systems.

These mosquitoes are likely to live more closely to people. Bites from some mosquitoes cause one of the world's biggest killers – **malaria**.

City killers

Many people are leaving the countryside for cities. There is not enough housing for everyone. Unplanned towns grow into slums on the edges of the city. There is often nowhere clean to wash or go to the toilet. People have little money for food.

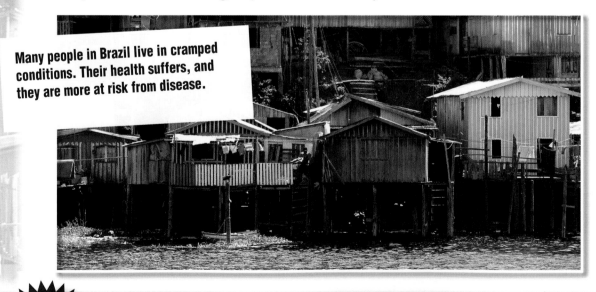

Many people in Brazil live in cramped conditions. Their health suffers, and they are more at risk from disease.

✦ In 2005, one in three people living in cities was housed in slum conditions.
✦ Around 1.1 million people live in the sprawling slums of Rio de Janeiro, Brazil.

People should move to the city: Who is right and who is wrong?

FOR

There is little work in rural areas, so people cannot afford to look after their families. **Climate change** is making it hard to grow crops because of extreme weather events that cause droughts and floods. There are more doctors in the city to help treat illnesses.

Many poor people living in cities such as Fianarantsoa in Madagascar rely on handouts. They cannot grow their own food.

AGAINST

Cities are **polluted** and dirty. There are very few places for children to play safely. People live so closely together that disease spreads quickly. Wouldn't it be better to make sure people can earn a good living in the countryside?

Too much wealth is bad for health

POVERTY CAUSES HEALTH problems. So too does wealth. Rich people are eating too much sugar and fat and taking less exercise. They are getting fatter. This is causing serious health problems.

Eating the wrong food

Many children are eating too much high-fat food with lots of sugar. This "junk" food is causing a health crisis, especially in the rich, **developed world**. Good food keeps your body and mind working. Without the essential **vitamins** and minerals from food, people are more likely to fall ill. Children cannot concentrate in class or miss school altogether.

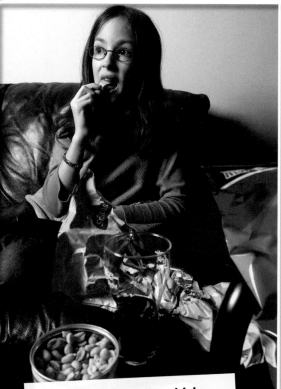

A diet of crisps and fizzy drinks combined with no exercise will lead to serious health problems.

Getting richer but not getting healthier

Many **developing countries** are becoming much richer. For example, India's economy is growing very quickly. In some parts of India, people are still very poor. Their health is suffering because of a lack of food and clean water.

In other parts of India, people are becoming richer. They have plenty of food and clean water. Rich people in India are facing new health problems. They are eating the wrong types of food and taking less exercise. They are beginning to suffer from health problems such as heart disease and other illnesses caused by being overweight.

BEHIND THE HEADLINES
Obese nation

The United States has one of the highest obesity rates in the world. More than 60 million adults and nine million children in the United States are considered to be obese. That's more than 60 per cent of the entire **population**. Obesity costs the country billions of dollars in medical care. Not only do many people in the United States eat too much of the wrong food, they also throw away a great deal of food and packaging. Much of it is dumped in landfill sites, which may in turn cause further health problems (see below).

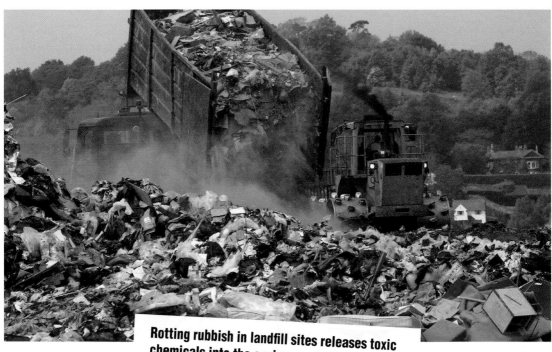

Rotting rubbish in landfill sites releases toxic chemicals into the environment. The rubbish also attracts pests that spread disease.

Emergency action to save lives

WILD WEATHER, DEVASTATING earthquakes, and terrible **tsunamis** – natural disasters are rarely out of the news. They cause major devastation, destroying homes and killing tens of thousands of people. Food shortages lead to **starvation**. Disease spreads as water supplies dry up and people start to drink dirty water. Dead bodies rot in the heat, attracting animals such as insects and rats. These pests also spread disease.

Climate change

The effects of pollution are changing weather around the world. Extreme weather events are all too common because of **climate change**. There are more droughts and floods.

Crops fail without rain. Without enough food, people starve. Land used to grow crops for food is now used to grow plants for **biofuels**. People are keen to use biofuels because they cause less pollution than **fossil fuels**. The world is getting hotter. This **global warming** is drying out once green and fertile land.

Safety or suffering?

Following a natural disaster or war, people often have to abandon their homes. They shelter in refugee camps. Thousands of people gather in these temporary camps. They live in cramped conditions, sharing small amounts of food and fresh water. Disease spreads quickly.

Earthquake survivors gather at a refugee camp in Anxian in Sichuan Province, China. Millions lost their homes in the disaster.

ON THE SPOT
Sichuan Province, China

On 12 May 2008, an earthquake hit Sichuan Province in China, causing devastation. Buildings collapsed, burying hundreds of thousands of people. The earthquake cut off electricity, so no one could cook or heat their homes – if the buildings were still standing.

There were no toilets and nowhere to wash. Water from burst drains and sewers ran freely in the streets. People ran the risk of catching diseases such as **cholera**, which spreads in such conditions. The clean-up operation took months, but it took much longer for people to rebuild their lives.

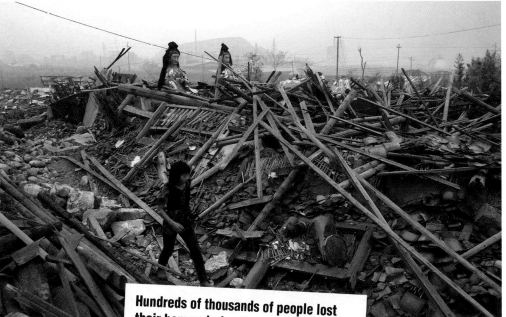

Hundreds of thousands of people lost their homes during the 2008 earthquake.

Medicine for all

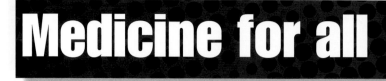

I F YOU ARE ill, you can go to see the doctor. He or she will give you medicine if you need it. In some parts of the world, people cannot afford to see a doctor. They often live in remote places, hours or even days away from the nearest medical centre. Illnesses that are easy to cure in one country may kill people in other parts of the world.

A dose of illness

People often say prevention is better than a cure. One way to prevent certain diseases is through **vaccines**. Vaccines are weak doses of a **bacterium** or **virus** that causes a disease. By giving someone the vaccine, the body builds up resistance to the disease. If the person comes into contact with the harmful **germ** again, they will not catch the disease.

Diseases such as measles used to kill thousands of children every year. Measles is caused by a virus. It can lead to blindness, brain damage, and even death. More and more children are now being vaccinated against this terrible disease. As a result, the number of children dying from measles has fallen dramatically.

All about money

Many doctors in the **developing world** do not have access to the drugs they need. Poor countries cannot afford to buy them. Instead, they want to make their own versions of the drugs. Then they could afford to give them to their own people.

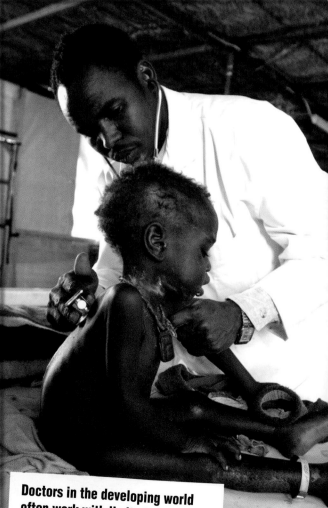

Doctors in the developing world often work with limited drugs and medical equipment.

Conventional medicine is better than alternative medicine:
Who is right and who is wrong?

FOR

Scientists test conventional medicines such as drugs. There are strict rules to make sure that the correct amount of a medicine is given. Doctors can warn people of any side effects. Drugs to cure illnesses such as **cholera** work. Alternative medicine uses methods such as homeopathy and herbal medicine. There is no scientific proof that alternative medicines work.

AGAINST

People have used alternative medicines such as herbal remedies for thousands of years. They are made from natural substances. Germs are beginning to resist many conventional drugs. This is creating more harmful types of diseases. Conventional drugs also cause side effects.

People place their trust in modern medicine even when it means having an injection.

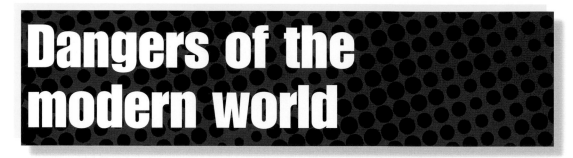

Dangers of the modern world

GERMS ARE SURVIVORS. Over time, they grow stronger and build up a resistance to drugs. These germs are called superbugs. MRSA is an example. It can cause illness and even death if it infects the blood. MRSA has built up a resistance to drugs called **antibiotics**.

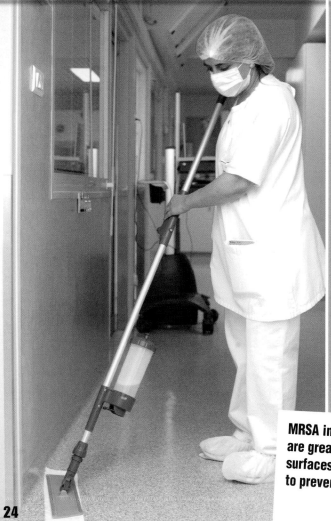

MRSA infects hospitals where people are greatly at risk from illness. Keeping surfaces clean and washing hands can help to prevent the spread of this superbug.

HIV and AIDS

Sometimes, a new disease appears for which there is no known cure. Human Immunodeficiency Virus (HIV) damages the immune system and causes other infections. The **virus** passes from person to person through body fluids such as blood and even breast milk. Over time, it can develop into the Acquired Immunodeficiency Syndrome (AIDS). There is no cure for AIDS, but there are drugs that can slow the development of HIV.

A new disease spreads across the world

In 2003, an American businessman died in a hospital in Vietnam. Doctors found out that he was infected with a virus called Severe Acute Respiratory Syndrome (SARS). Doctors think that the virus came from China. Roughly 800 people have died due to SARS. So far there is no known cure for the deadly disease.

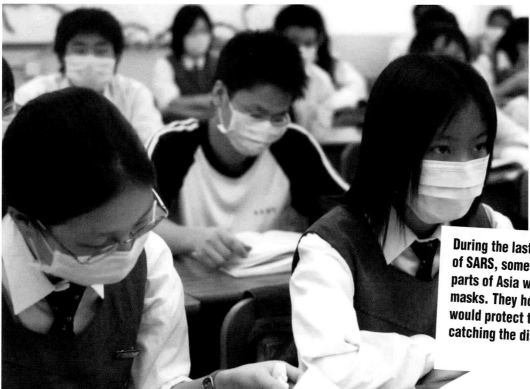

During the last outbreak of SARS, some people in parts of Asia wore face masks. They hoped this would protect them from catching the disease.

ON THE SPOT
South Africa

Today, people in South Africa are facing an **epidemic** of HIV infection. Millions of people are dying from this disease. By the end of 2005, over 15 million children had lost their parents to AIDS.

Hundreds of thousands more were infected with HIV themselves. Not everyone can afford drugs that slow down the HIV virus. People are learning more about HIV so that they do not pass on the disease.

Take control for a healthy future

THERE ARE NOW nearly seven billion people living on Earth. The **population** is growing every day. Advances in medicine help people to live longer. As people grow older, however, they are likely to develop new health problems, which need new medical solutions. It is a constant struggle to keep the world in good health.

Knowledge is health

Health programmes have been set up around the world to teach people about the health issues they are facing. Organizations working in the **developing world** provide people with the knowledge to live healthier lives. They are helping local communities to build fresh, clean water supplies and clean toilet facilities.

Polluted air

Whenever you drive in a car, play a computer game, watch television, or switch on a light you are using electricity. This energy is produced by burning **fossil fuels** such as coal, natural gas, and oil. When fossil fuels burn, they produce lots of smoke and gas, which **pollutes** the air. Breathing in polluted air can cause serious health problems, such as **asthma** and other respiratory conditions. For our future people must try to find cleaner ways to generate electricity.

Many children suffer from asthma, particularly in polluted city centres.

Everyone has the right to medical care: Who is right and who is wrong?

Many people are aware that eating too many fatty foods, smoking, and drinking too much alcohol can lead to poor health. Should doctors spend time treating people with illnesses caused by their own poor lifestyle choices?

FOR

If alcohol, cigarettes, and fatty foods are so damaging to our health, why are people still allowed to buy them? Governments cannot allow these unhealthy products to be sold and then refuse people medical care when they become ill.

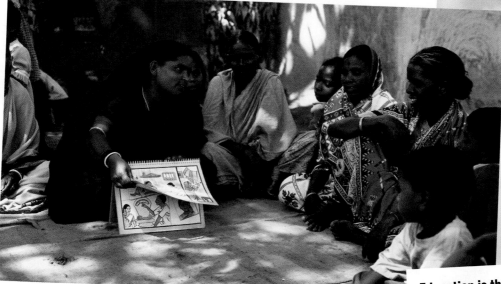

Education is the key to helping people live healthier lives.

AGAINST

People should take responsibility for their own health. People know that smoking is harmful. If they become unwell, they are to blame. Doctors should not waste their time and effort on people who choose an unhealthy lifestyle.

27

Get involved!

Most people can try to stay fit and healthy by eating good food and taking lots of exercise. We can also help other people who are less fortunate so they can enjoy healthy lives, too.

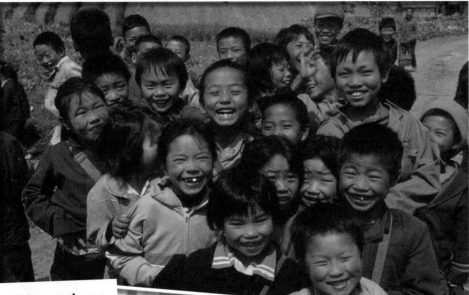

Healthy children are happy children who can go to school and learn how to make better lives for themselves and others.

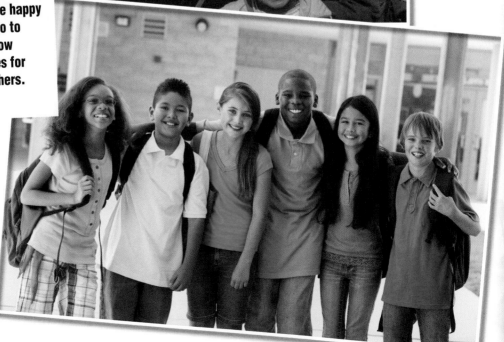

THINGS TO DO

Eat well

- Eat foods that provide the goodness the body needs to stay healthy. These nutrients include carbohydrates, proteins, vitamins, minerals, and a small amount of fats.

Stay clean

- Always wash your hands after going to the toilet. Always wash your hands before eating.
- Make sure food is properly prepared and cooked.
- Wash fruit and vegetables in clean, fresh water.

Get involved

- Many **charities** work to help reduce **poverty** and improve the health of people in **developing countries**. Organize a fun run or a quiz to raise money for your chosen **charity**.

School swap

- Find out about schools in a developing country. What are the different health issues that affect school children in another part of the world?

Get moving

- Take regular exercise to keep your heart and lungs working well. Regular exercise keeps you fit and feeling good.

Save energy

- The amount, and type, of energy that we use has an effect on the health of people around the world. Pollution from burning **fossil fuels** poisons the air.
- Investigate the different types of energy sources you could use at home or school. Could your school install solar panels to capture the Sun's power? Could solar energy be used instead of the electricity from fossil fuels?
- Avoid travelling by car as much as possible. Ride a bike to school instead of getting a lift. This will help reduce pollution and slow down **climate change**.

Dangers

- Be aware of the dangers of smoking, drinking alcohol, and taking illegal drugs.

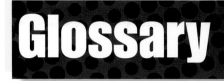

Glossary

antibiotic drug used to treat bacteria that cause diseases

asthma condition that causes a person's airways to narrow, which makes it difficult for them to breathe

bacterium tiny cell. Some bacteria are healthy but some cause disease.

biofuel fuel made from plants such as palm oil seeds and sugar cane

cancer serious illness caused by a tumour (growth) in part of the body

cell tiny structure that makes up all the different parts of the body

charity organization that collects money and uses it to help good causes

cholera disease carried in polluted water. It affects the digestive system and can cause death if left untreated.

climate change changes in the world's weather patterns caused by human activities. These include burning fossil fuels, such as oil and coal, which cause pollution and release harmful gases into the atmosphere.

communicable disease disease that can pass from person to person either directly or by a host such as an insect

crop plant grown by farmers

dehydrated having lost too much water

developed country rich country

developing country poor country

environment your surroundings

epidemic when a disease spreads quickly among many people

fossil fuel fuel made from animals and plants that grew millions of years ago

germ tiny bacterium or virus that lives in plants and animals

global warming increase in the average temperature at Earth's surface

immune system body's natural defence against germs

infectious spread from one living thing to another

insecticide chemical that kills insects

malaria infectious disease caused by tiny germs that are spread through the bites of some types of mosquitoes

malnutrition not having enough goodness from food to keep the body healthy

microscope tool that allows people to look at tiny objects that cannot be seen by the naked human eye

pollute make dirty

population the number of people in a given area

poverty not having enough money for basic things such as food and shelter

prescribe to give a patient a particular drug or medicine

sewage all the liquid and solid waste material from toilets and sinks, which is carried away by drains and sewers

starvation state of extreme hunger resulting from lack of essential nutrients over a long period

tsunami giant ocean wave caused by earthquakes on the ocean floor

vaccine small dose of a virus. It is given to a person to help prevent him or her catching the disease.

virus type of germ that causes illness

vitamin substance the body needs in tiny amounts to stay healthy

Find out more

Books

Am I Fit and Healthy?: Learning About Diet and Exercise (Me And My Body), Claire Llewellyn (Hodder Wayland, 2007)

Epidemics (In The News), Ann Kramer (Franklin Watts, 2006)

Exercise (It's Your Health), Beverley Goodger (Franklin Watts, 2004)

Food for Feeling Healthy (Making Healthy Food Choices), Carol Ballard (Heinemann Library, 2007)

Health and Disease (Planet Under Pressure), Claire Wallerstein (Heinemann Library, 2007)

Nice or Nasty?: Learning About Drugs and Your Health (Me And My Body), Claire Llewellyn (Hodder Wayland, 2007)

Obesity and Health (In The News), Adam Hibbert (Franklin Watts, 2005)

Websites

This site looks at the health problems associated with eating too much or too little food and talks about some of the ways in which we can live healthier lives:
www.actionforhealthykids.org/

This website is packed with excellent articles about health issues. "The Game Closet" activity section includes lots of fun games and experiments. Go to:
www.kidshealth.org/kid

This website lists articles in order of subject. Click on the "Health and Pollution" link to find out more information about the price of pollution on human health at:
www.peopleandplanet.net/

Index